Thriving as a New Nurse: A Practical Guide to Confidence, Safe Practice, and Staying Sane

Alice Ashu

Author's Note

Growing into the Nurse You're Meant to Be

When I first stepped into nursing, I didn't feel confident. I didn't feel strong. I didn't feel like the kind of person who could walk into a patient's room and speak with authority. I was an immigrant in a new country, far from the small community where I grew up, and even farther from anything that felt familiar or safe.

I worried about everything: my accent, my soft voice, my shyness, my ability to fit into a profession where everyone seemed so sure of themselves. I often wondered if anyone standing next to me could even hear me speak. It wasn't that my voice was naturally quiet; it was that I didn't yet believe in myself enough to speak with confidence.

But something unexpected happened. The people around me, my clinical preceptors, my instructors, my early mentors, saw something in me long before I saw it myself. They noticed my passion, my curiosity, my compassion. They told me I would be an extraordinary nurse, even when I still felt like I was trying to find my footing.

During my new-grad orientation, I was paired with a preceptor I admired deeply. She was knowledgeable, confident, and experienced. Everything I thought I wasn't. Yet she trusted me early. She let me take on tasks sooner than I expected because she said I had strong critical thinking and a natural ability to build trust with patients. Her belief in me became the foundation I didn't know I needed.

And then there were my patients, the true teachers of my nursing journey.

I remember one young woman I cared for over three nights. She was scared, overwhelmed, and facing surgery; she didn't fully understand. I was with her before the procedure, the night of her surgery, and the day after. On my last morning with her, she held my hand, tears in her eyes, and told me she believed God had sent me to her. She said my calm spirit and softness kept her going.

For so long, I thought being calm was a flaw. I thought being soft- spoken meant I wasn't strong enough for nursing. But my patients taught me otherwise. They showed me that calm is a gift. Softness is a strength. Compassion is a skill.

Even my first nurse manager, who left her position months into my career, still reaches out to check on me. She once wrote to me, "You have that compassion that some people lack. Always remember we are doing God's work as we help our patients. You are blessed. Never forget that." Her words still stay with me.

My confidence didn't come all at once. It grew slowly, through moments like these, moments of connection, trust, and quiet courage. And that's why I wrote this book.

Because I know what it feels like to doubt yourself.

I know what it feels like to wonder if you belong.

I know what it feels like to be new, overwhelmed, and unsure.

But I also know this:

If I could grow into the nurse I am today, confident, capable, trusted, and proud, then you can grow into the nurse you're meant to be, too.

This book is not about perfection. It's about growth.

It's about learning to think critically, practice safely, and care for yourself as much as you care for your patients.

It's about finding your voice, even if it starts out soft.

It's about thriving, not just surviving, in your first year and beyond.

Wherever you are in your journey, scared, excited, overwhelmed, hopeful, I'm here with you. And I'm cheering for you.

Introduction

You Are Not Alone in This Journey

Your first year as a nurse will change you in ways you can't fully imagine yet. It will challenge you, stretch you, and teach you lessons that no classroom, no textbook, and no simulation lab could ever prepare you for. It will also shape you, strengthen you, and reveal a version of yourself you haven't met yet, a version that is capable, resilient, compassionate, and steady.

But before all of that happens, there's a moment every new nurse faces:

The moment you step onto the unit for the first time and feel the weight of responsibility settle onto your shoulders.

Maybe you're excited.

Maybe you're nervous.

Maybe you're overwhelmed.

Maybe you're all three at once.

If so, you're exactly where you're supposed to be.

This book was written for you, the new nurse who wants to do well, who wants to feel confident, who wants to make a difference, but who may also feel unsure, anxious, or out of place. You're not alone in those feelings. Every nurse you admire has stood exactly where you are now, wondering if they were ready, wondering if they would ever feel confident, wondering if they belonged.

You do belong.

And you will grow into this role.

Why I Wrote This Book

Nursing school teaches you the foundation, but your first year teaches you how to be a nurse. It teaches you how to think, how to communicate, how to prioritize, how to stay calm under pressure, and how to care for yourself while caring for others.

But too often, new nurses feel like they're supposed to figure everything out on their own. They feel like they're the only ones struggling, the only ones overwhelmed, the only ones who don't feel confident yet.

You're not the only one.

You're not behind.

You're not failing.

You're learning.

This book exists to guide you through that learning, with honesty, compassion, and practical wisdom.

This Book Explores

This is not a textbook.

This is not a lecture.

This is not a list of impossible expectations.

This is a guide written with you in mind, the real you, the human you, the new nurse who is trying their best.

Here, you'll discover:

- Reassurance for the moments you feel overwhelmed
- Practical tools for staying safe and organized
- Strategies for communication, time management, and clinical

Judgment

- Guidance for handling stress and preventing burnout
- Encouragement as you grow into your professional identity

Each chapter is designed to meet you where you are and help you take the next step with confidence.

A Note from One Nurse to Another

You don't have to be perfect to be a great nurse.

You don't have to know everything to be safe.

You don't have to feel confident to show up with compassion.

You just have to keep learning, keep asking questions, and keep caring, even on the hard days.

Your first year will challenge you, but it will also shape you into the nurse you're meant to be. And you don't have to walk that journey alone. This book is here to support you, steady you, and remind you of your strength every step of the way.

Take a deep breath.

You're ready for this even if you don't feel ready yet.

Let's begin.

Contents

Author's Note...v

Introduction...ix

Why I Wrote This Book...xi

A Note from One Nurse to Another xiii

Chapter 1 If You Feel Out of Place, You're Not Alone 1

Chapter 2 Understanding the Hospital Ecosystem.............................5

Chapter 3 Building Real Clinical Judgment....................................12

Chapter 4 Safe Practice Essentials 18

Chapter 5 Time Management for New Nurses...................................24

Chapter 6 Communicating with Confidence....................................30

Chapter 7 Handling Stressful Situations 35

Chapter 8 Preventing Burnout Before It Starts 40

Chapter 9 Growing into Your Professional Identity..........................46

Chapter 10 Becoming the Nurse You're Meant to Be.........................51

Closing Thoughts 55

About the Author..57

Chapter 1 If You Feel Out of Place, You're Not Alone

The first days and weeks of being a new nurse can feel like stepping into a world where everyone else seems to know exactly what they're doing. You look around and see nurses moving with confidence, speaking with certainty, and handling situations that still make your heart race. It's easy to wonder if you're the only one who feels unsure, overwhelmed, or out of place.

You're not.

Feeling out of place is one of the most universal experiences in nursing. It doesn't mean you're unprepared. It doesn't mean you're not smart enough. And it definitely doesn't mean you chose the wrong profession. It simply means you're new, and being new at something this complex takes time, patience, and grace.

The Myth of the "Naturally Confident Nurse"

Many new nurses assume confidence is something you're supposed to walk in with on day one. But confidence in nursing isn't a personality trait; it's a skill. It's built through repetition, exposure, mistakes, questions, and moments of growth that happen quietly over time.

The nurses who look confident today weren't always that way. They had shaky hands, racing thoughts, and moments where they questioned everything. They learned, shift by shift, that confidence grows from showing up, trying again, and allowing themselves to be beginners.

You Belong Here, Even If You Don't Feel Like it Yet

It's normal to feel like you're behind everyone else. It's normal to feel intimidated by the pace, the responsibilities, and the expectations. But belonging isn't something you earn by being perfect. It's something you grow into by being present, willing, and committed.

You belong here because:

- You care about people
- You're willing to learn
- You show up even when you're nervous
- You're trying, even when it feels hard

Those qualities matter far more than sounding confident or looking experienced.

Growth Happens Quietly

Confidence doesn't arrive in a dramatic moment. It builds slowly, often without you noticing. One day, you'll realize you didn't second- guess yourself as much. You'll catch yourself explaining something clearly to a patient.

You'll handle a situation that once terrified you. You'll speak up without rehearsing the words in your head first.

These small shifts are the real markers of growth. They're subtle, but they're powerful.

It's Okay to Ask Questions, In Fact, It's Necessary

New nurses sometimes worry that asking questions makes them look unprepared. The truth is the opposite. Asking questions shows awareness, responsibility, and a commitment to safe practice. It's how you learn. It's how you protect your patients. It's how you build trust with your team.

Experienced nurses don't expect you to know everything. They expect you to care enough to ask.

Your Strengths Might Not Look Like Everyone Else's

Some nurses are loud and assertive. Some are calm and steady. Some are analytical. Some are intuitive. Some lead with humor. Some lead with gentleness.

There is no single "right" way to be a nurse.

Your strengths, even the ones you don't fully recognize yet, will shape the kind of nurse you become. And your patients will appreciate you for exactly who you are.

Give Yourself Permission to Grow

You don't have to be confident today. You don't have to know everything. You don't have to match anyone else's pace. You just have to keep showing up, learning, asking, and trying.

Confidence will come.

Skill will come.

Comfort will come.

Belonging will come.

You're not behind. You're not failing. You're not alone.

You're simply growing, and growth takes time.

This chapter is your reminder that you're in the right place. You're becoming the nurse you're meant to be, even if you can't see it yet. And every shift, every question, every challenge is shaping you into someone stronger, wiser, and more confident than you realize.

You're not out of place.

You're just at the beginning.

And beginnings are supposed to feel unfamiliar.

Chapter 2 Understanding the Hospital Ecosystem

Stepping into a hospital as a new nurse can feel like entering a small city, one with its own language, culture, rhythm, and unspoken rules. It's busy, fast- moving, and full of people who seem to know exactly where they're going and what they're doing. But the truth is, every nurse, doctor, technician, and staff member you see once stood exactly where you are now: trying to make sense of it all.

Understanding the hospital ecosystem is one of the first steps toward feeling grounded and confident in your role. When you know how the system works, you can navigate it with more ease, communicate more effectively, and build stronger relationships with the people around you.

This chapter will help you understand the environment you're stepping into, not just the tasks, but the culture, the teamwork, and the flow that make a hospital function.

The Hospital Is a Team Sport

Nursing is not a solo profession. You're a part of a team, a large, interconnected one, and every role matters. When you understand who does what, you'll feel less pressure to do everything yourself and more confident in asking for help when you need it.

Here are some of the key players you'll interact with:

Charge Nurse

The charge nurse oversees the unit for the shift. They:

- Assign patient loads
- Help troubleshoot problems
- Coordinate admissions, discharges, and transfers
- Support the team when things get busy

They're your go- to person when you're unsure about something or need guidance.

Nurse Manager

The nurse manager handles the bigger picture:

- Staffing
- Scheduling
- Unit policies
- Performance evaluations

You may not interact with them as often, but they play a major role in shaping the unit culture.

Certified Nursing Assistants (CNAs) or Patient Care Technicians

Your CNAs are essential partners. They assist with:

- Vital signs

- Hygiene care
- Ambulation
- Blood glucose checks
- Basic patient needs

A strong relationship with your CNAs will make your shifts smoother and your patients better cared for.

Physicians and Advanced Practice Providers

These include:

- Residents
- Attendings
- Nurse practitioners
- Physician assistants

Your role is to communicate clearly, advocate for your patients, and collaborate on care plans.

Ancillary Staff

These are the behind- the- scenes heroes:

- Respiratory therapists
- Physical and occupational therapists
- Pharmacists
- Case managers
- Social workers
- Dietary staff
- Environmental services

Knowing who to call and when will save you time and reduce stress.

Every Unit Has Its Own Culture

Even within the same hospital, each unit has its own personality. Some are fast- paced and loud. Others are calm and structured. Some teams joke around. Others are more serious. Some units feel like family. Others feel more formal.

As a new nurse, you're learning not just the tasks, but the culture. Pay attention to:

- How nurses communicate with each other
- How they handle stress
- How they support one another
- How they interact with leadership
- How they approach patient care

You don't have to change who you are to fit in. You simply learn how the team works and find your place within it.

The Flow of a Shift

Understanding the rhythm of a shift helps you feel more prepared and less overwhelmed. While every unit is different, most shifts follow a similar pattern:

1. Shift Report

This is where you get the story of your patients. Listen closely, ask questions, and take notes in a way that works for you.

2. First Rounds

You'll assess your patients, check orders, and prioritize your tasks. This sets the tone for your shift.

3. Med Passes and Treatments

Medication administration, wound care, blood sugars, and other routine tasks fill much of your time.

4. Charting

Documentation is essential. Chart as you go when possible; it reduces stress later.

5. Admissions, Discharges, and Transfers

These can happen at any time and often shift your priorities quickly.

6. Ongoing Monitoring

You'll respond to call lights, reassess patients, communicate with providers, and adjust care plans as needed.

7. End- of- Shift Wrap- Up

Finish charting, tie up loose ends, and give a thorough report to the next nurse.

The more familiar you become with this flow, the more confident and organized you'll feel.

Communication Is Your Superpower

Clear communication is one of the most important skills you'll develop. It helps you:

- Advocate for your patients
- Build trust with your team
- Prevent errors
- Stay organized
- Feel more confident

You don't need to speak loudly to communicate effectively. You just need to speak clearly, respectfully, and with intention.

You Don't Have to Know Everything. You Just Have to Know How to Navigate

No one expects you to understand the entire hospital ecosystem on day one. Or day ten. Or even day one hundred. What matters is that you're learning, observing, asking questions, and slowly building your understanding.

Over time, the hospital will feel less like a maze and more like a familiar environment. You'll know who to call, where to go, how to prioritize, and how to work with your team. You'll move with more confidence because you'll understand the system you're a part of.

You're not supposed to know everything yet.

You're supposed to grow into it.

And you will.

Chapter 3 Building Real Clinical Judgment

One of the biggest transitions from nursing school to bedside nursing is learning how to think like a nurse. Not just follow steps, but make decisions, anticipate needs, and understand the "why" behind everything you do. This ability is called clinical judgment, and it's the foundation of a safe, confident nursing practice.

The good news is that clinical judgment is not something you're expected to master on day one. It's something you build, layer by layer, through experience, observation, and reflection. This chapter will help you understand what clinical judgment really means and how to strengthen it as a new nurse.

Clinical Judgment Is More Than Knowledge

In school, you learned facts, skills, and procedures. At the bedside, you learn how to apply them in real time, with real patients, in situations that don't always look like the textbook.

Clinical judgment involves:

- Recognizing what's important
- Understanding what could go wrong

- Prioritizing what needs to be done first
- Knowing when to ask for help
- Anticipating changes before they happen

It's not about being perfect. It's about being aware, thoughtful, and willing to learn.

Start with the Basics: What's Normal and What's Not

You can't recognize a problem if you don't know what normal looks like. As a new nurse, one of the most valuable habits you can build is learning your patient's baseline.

Ask yourself:

- What are their vital signs normally like
- How do they look when they're stable
- What is their mental status
- How do they breathe
- What is their pain level
- What is their mobility

When you know your patient's baseline, you'll notice subtle changes sooner, and early recognition is one of the strongest signs of good clinical judgment.

Use Frameworks to Guide Your Thinking

When you're new, it's easy to feel overwhelmed by everything happening at once. Frameworks help you organize your thoughts and make safe decisions.

Some of the most helpful include:

ABCs: Airway, Breathing, Circulation

Always start here. If any of these are compromised, they become your top priority.

Maslow's Hierarchy of Needs.

Physiological needs (breathing, circulation, pain, elimination) come before emotional or educational needs.

Safety First.

Ask yourself:

What could harm this patient if I don't address it now?

Acute vs. Chronic

Acute changes usually require faster intervention than chronic conditions.

These frameworks don't replace your judgment; they support it.

Pay Attention to Patterns

Over time, you'll start to notice patterns:

- Certain symptoms often appear together
- Certain medications have predictable side effects
- Certain diagnoses follow a typical progression

- Certain lab values hint at what might happen next

Pattern recognition is a major part of clinical judgment, and it grows naturally with experience. Don't rush it. Let it develop as you care for more patients and encounter more situations.

Ask "Why" Constantly

One of the strongest habits you can build is asking yourself:

- Why is this happening?
- Why was this medication ordered?
- Why is this lab value important?
- Why is the provider concerned about this symptom?

The more you understand the "why," the more confident you'll feel, and the safer your practice will be.

Know When to Ask for Help

Good clinical judgment isn't about doing everything alone. It's about knowing when something doesn't feel right and speaking up.

You should ask for help when:

- A patient looks different from before
- You're unsure if a symptom is concerning
- You're uncomfortable performing a task alone
- You feel overwhelmed

- You sense something is wrong, but can't explain it yet

Experienced nurses don't expect you to know everything. They expect you to care enough to ask.

Trust Your Observations

As a new nurse, you might doubt yourself. You might think, maybe I'm overreacting. But if something feels off, pay attention. Nurses often notice subtle changes long before the monitors or labs show anything.

Your instincts will sharpen with time, but even now, they matter.

Reflect After Every Shift

Reflection is one of the most powerful tools for building clinical judgment. After each shift, ask yourself:

- What went well
- What challenged me
- What did I learn
- What would I do differently next time

Reflection turns experience into wisdom.

Clinical Judgment Grows with You

You don't build clinical judgment by memorizing facts. You build it by:

- Showing up
- Paying attention
- Asking questions
- Learning from mistakes
- Reflecting on your experiences
- Caring deeply about your patients

Every shift strengthens your judgment. Every patient teaches you something new. Every challenge shapes you into a more confident, capable nurse.

You're not expected to know everything right now. You're expected to grow, and you are.

Chapter 4 Safe Practice Essentials

One of the most important responsibilities you carry as a nurse is keeping your patients safe. Safety isn't just a checklist; it's a mindset. It's the way you approach your work, the way you think through decisions, and the way you protect your patients, your license, and yourself.

As a new nurse, it's normal to feel nervous about making mistakes. That fear doesn't mean you're unprepared; it means you care. And caring is the foundation of safe practice. Over time, your confidence will grow, but safety will always remain at the center of everything you do.

This chapter will guide you through the core principles of safe nursing practice so you can step into each shift with clarity and assurance.

Safety Starts with Awareness

Safe practice begins with being aware of your patients, your environment, your limitations, and your responsibilities. Awareness helps you catch small issues before they become big problems.

Ask yourself throughout your shift:

- What am I seeing
- What am I hearing
- What is changing
- What needs my attention first

Being present and observant is one of the strongest safety tools you have.

Medication Safety: Slow Down to Stay Safe

Medication administration is one of the highest- risk areas for new nurses. The best way to stay safe is to slow down, even when the unit feels fast.

Keep these principles close:

The Rights of Medication Administration

You learned them in school, but now they matter more than ever:

- Right patient
- Right medication
- Right dose
- Right route
- Right time
- Right documentation
- Right reason
- Right response

Never rush through these steps. Your patients depend on your attention to detail.

Double- Check High- Risk Medications

Insulin, anticoagulants, opioids, electrolytes, and certain IV drips require extra caution. If your facility requires a second nurse to verify, take that seriously; it's there to protect your patient and your license.

Trust Your Instincts

If something feels off, a dose seems too high, an order doesn't match the patient's condition, or a medication looks unfamiliar, pause and verify. Asking questions is a sign of safe practice, not weakness.

Documentation Protects You and Your Patients

Charting isn't just a task; it's a legal record of your care. Clear, accurate documentation:

- Supports continuity of care
- Protects you in case of questions or audits
- Helps providers make informed decisions
- Reflects your professionalism

Chart as You Go

Waiting until the end of your shift increases the risk of forgetting important details. Even brief notes throughout the shift help you stay accurate.

Be Objective and Specific

Instead of:

- "Anxious patient."

Try:

- "Patient pacing room, breathing fast, stating 'I feel nervous.'"

Specific details paint a clearer picture and reduce misunderstandings.

Know Your Scope and Respect It

Every nurse has a defined scope of practice based on their license and facility policies. Staying within your scope is essential for safe practice.

This means:

- Don't perform procedures you haven't been trained or validated to do
- Don't guess, verify
- Don't let anyone pressure you into doing something unsafe

Your license is your responsibility. Protect it.

Delegation: You Don't Have to Do Everything Yourself

Delegation is a skill that takes time to develop. It's not about handing off tasks; it's about ensuring the right person does the right job safely.

When delegating to CNAs or techs:

- Be clear about what you need
- Provide important patient details
- Follow up to ensure completion
- Show appreciation for their work

Delegation helps you stay organized and ensures your patients receive timely care.

Preventing Common New- Grad Mistakes

Every new nurse makes mistakes; it's part of learning. But many common errors can be prevented with awareness and good habits.

Here are a few to watch for:

1. Rushing

Hurrying leads to missed steps. Slow down when it matters most.

2. Not Asking Questions

If you're unsure, ask. Silence is riskier than curiosity.

3. Skipping Reassessments

Patients can change quickly. Reassess after interventions, medications, or concerning symptoms.

4. Overlooking Subtle Changes

A slight change in mental status, breathing pattern, or skin color can be the first sign of deterioration.

5. Not Speaking Up

If something doesn't feel right, say something. Your voice matters.

Safety Is a Habit, Not A Skill

Safe practice isn't something you master once; it's something you commit to every day. It's built through:

- Consistency
- Attention to detail
- Asking questions
- Staying humble
- Staying curious

You don't have to be perfect to be safe. You just have to be intentional.

Over time, these habits will become second nature. You'll move with more confidence, make decisions with more clarity, and trust yourself more deeply. Safe practice is the foundation of great nursing, and you're already building it, one shift at a time.

Chapter 5 Time Management for New Nurses

Time management is one of the most challenging skills for new nurses and one of the most transformative once you begin to develop it. In the beginning, it may feel like the shift is moving faster than you can keep up. Tasks pile up, call lights ring, charting waits, and you may wonder how experienced nurses make it all look so effortless.

The truth is, they didn't start out that way. Time management is learned through practice, patience, and a willingness to grow. This chapter will help you build a realistic, flexible approach to managing your time so you can stay organized, reduce stress, and provide safe, compassionate care.

Time Management Begins with Prioritization

You cannot do everything at once, and you're not supposed to. Prioritization is the foundation of effective time management.

A helpful way to think about your tasks is to sort them into four categories:

- Urgent: Needs immediate attention to protect life or safety
- Important: Supports patient stability and comfort
- Routine: Necessary tasks that can be scheduled
- Delegable: Tasks that can be safely assigned to CNAs or techs

When you learn to separate what needs to happen now from what can happen later, your shift becomes clearer and more manageable.

Start Your Shift with a Realistic Plan

The first hour of your shift sets the tone for everything that follows. A strong start helps you stay ahead instead of constantly catching up.

1. **Get the Report and Do It at the Bedside Whenever Possible**

In a perfect world, every report would be thorough, organized, and complete. In real life, that's not always the case. The outgoing nurse may have had a difficult shift, may be overwhelmed, or may not have had time to review every detail.

But one thing you can control is where you receive the report.

Whenever possible, do your report at the bedside, not at the nurses' station, not in the hallway, and not standing by the door.

Bedside report allows you to:

- Lay eyes on your patient immediately
- Confirm their identity
- Observe their breathing, color, and overall appearance
- Check IV lines, drains, wounds, and equipment
- Notice anything the outgoing nurse may have missed
- Build trust with your patient from the very start

Standing at the door or relying only on verbal report increases the risk of missing important details. A patient can look completely different from how they were described, and you won't know unless you see them.

If the outgoing nurse tries to give a report away from the bedside, you can gently say something like:

- "Let's step in so I can see the patient while we talk."
- "It helps me start my shift safely if I can lay eyes on them."

This isn't being demanding; it's practicing safe nursing.

2. Verify with the Chart

After the bedside report, take a few minutes to confirm the details:

- Review orders
- Scan recent provider notes
- Check labs and imaging
- Look at the MAR

This step helps you fill in any gaps and start your shift with accurate information.

3. Do Quick First Rounds

Even after the bedside report, do your own brief assessments. This helps you identify who needs attention first and gives you a baseline for the rest of your shift.

4. Build a Simple Timeline

Ask yourself:

- What needs to happen now
- What needs to happen in the next few hours
- What can wait

- What can be delegated

A plan doesn't have to be perfect; it just needs to guide you.

Cluster Your Care

Running in and out of rooms during your entire shift drains your time and energy. Clustering care helps you work efficiently while still providing excellent care.

For example:

- Bring medications, supplies, and equipment with you
- Combine assessments with medication passes
- Address multiple needs in one visit

Clustering care isn't rushing; it's being intentional.

Chart as You Go

Saving all your charting for the end of the shift is one of the biggest time traps for new nurses. It leads to stress, incomplete documentation, and the risk of forgetting important details.

Instead:

- Chart after each major task or assessment
- Use small pockets of downtime
- Keep brief notes if you can't chart immediately

Your documentation will be more accurate, and your shift will feel more manageable.

Use Your Team Wisely

You are not meant to do everything alone. CNAs, techs, charge nurses, and other team members are there to support you.

Delegate tasks such as:

- Vital signs
- Blood sugars
- Ambulation
- Hygiene care
- Bed changes

Delegation is not a sign of weakness; it's a sign of safe, effective nursing.

Expect the Unexpected

Even the best- planned shift can change in an instant. A patient may deteriorate. A new admission may arrive. A procedure may be delayed. A medication may be missing.

When this happens:

- Pause
- Reassess your priorities
- Adjust your plan
- Communicate with your team

Flexibility is a major part of time management.

Give Yourself Grace

Time management is one of the hardest skills for new nurses. You will have shifts where you feel behind. You will have days where nothing goes as planned. You will have moments where you question whether you're cut out for this.

But with each shift, you'll get better. You'll move more confidently. You'll anticipate needs sooner. You'll find your rhythm.

Time management isn't about perfection; it's about progress.

And you're already moving in the right direction.

Chapter 6 Communicating with Confidence

Communication is one of the most powerful tools you have as a nurse. It shapes your relationships with patients, builds trust with your team, and protects your patients' safety. Yet for many new nurses, communication is also one of the most intimidating parts of the job.

You may worry about sounding inexperienced.

You may feel nervous speaking to providers.

You may hesitate to ask questions.

You may fear being judged for not knowing something.

These feelings are normal, and they do not mean you're unprepared. They simply mean you're new. Confidence in communication grows with time, practice, and experience. This chapter will help you build the foundation you need to speak clearly, advocate effectively, and feel more grounded in your role.

Communication is a Skill, Not a Personality Trait

You don't have to be loud, extroverted, or outspoken to communicate well. Effective communication is about clarity, respect, and intention, not volume.

Some of the strongest communicators in nursing are calm, soft- spoken, and thoughtful. What matters is that your message is clear and your purpose is steady.

Start With Clarity

When you communicate with your team, aim to be:

- Clear
- Direct
- Concise
- Respectful

You don't need long explanations or complicated language. Simple, focused communication is often the safest and most effective.

For example, instead of:

- "I'm not sure, but I think maybe the patient might be having some trouble breathing."

Try:

- "The patient's breathing has changed. Respirations increased from 16 to 28, and they look more distressed."

Clarity builds trust, and it helps your team respond quickly.

Use Structured Communication Tools

Many hospitals use communication frameworks to help nurses speak clearly and confidently. One of the most common is SBAR:

- S, Situation: What is happening right now
- B, Background: Relevant history or context
- A, Assessment: What you think is going on
- R, Recommendation: What you need or suggest

SBAR helps you stay organized, especially when speaking to providers.

For example:

"This is the nurse on 4 West. I'm calling about Mr. Lopez in room 412. His blood pressure dropped from 118/72 to 86/50 in the last hour. He's pale and dizzy. I recommend evaluating him for possible fluid bolus or medication adjustment."

Structured communication makes you sound confident even when you're still learning.

Asking Questions Is a Sign of Strength

New nurses often hesitate to ask questions because they fear looking inexperienced. But asking questions is one of the most responsible things you can do.

Ask when:

- You're unsure about an order
- You don't understand a medication
- A patient's condition doesn't make sense
- You feel something is unsafe
- You need clarification

Experienced nurses don't expect you to know everything. They expect you to care enough to ask.

Advocating for Your Patients

Advocacy is one of your most important roles. Sometimes you'll be the first person to notice a change. Sometimes you'll be the only one who sees a risk. Speaking up can feel intimidating, but your voice matters.

Advocacy can sound like:

- "I understand the plan, but the patient is still in significant pain."
- "I'm concerned about this change in mental status."
- "This doesn't seem like their baseline."
- "I don't feel comfortable giving this medication without clarification."

You are not being difficult; you are protecting your patient.

Communicating with Difficult Personalities

You will encounter providers, nurses, or staff members who communicate in ways that feel abrupt, rushed, or dismissive. This is part of the hospital environment, not a reflection of your worth or competence.

When faced with difficult communication:

- Stay calm
- Stay factual
- Stay focused on the patient
- Don't take it personally

You can be firm and respectful at the same time.

For example:

- "I hear your concern. Here's what I'm seeing with the patient."
- "I want to make sure we're on the same page for safety."

Your professionalism speaks louder than their tone.

Communicating with Patients and Families

Patients and families often feel scared, confused, or overwhelmed. Your communication can bring them comfort and clarity.

Aim to:

- Speak slowly and calmly
- Use simple language
- Listen without interrupting
- Validate their feelings
- Be honest about what you know and don't know. You don't need all the answers. You just need to be present.

Confidence Comes with Practice

You won't feel confident in every conversation, and that's okay. Confidence grows through:

- Repetition
- Experience
- Observation
- Reflection
- Support from your team

Every shift strengthens your communication skills. Every conversation teaches you something new. Every moment you speak up, even when your voice shakes, builds your confidence.

You don't have to communicate perfectly.

You just have to communicate with intention.

And you're already doing that.

Chapter 7 Handling Stressful Situations

No matter how prepared you are, nursing will place you in stressful situations. A patient may deteriorate suddenly. A family member may become emotional. A provider may be rushed. Your unit may be short- staffed. You may feel pulled in ten different directions at once.

Feeling stressed doesn't mean you're failing; it means you're human.

And learning how to stay grounded in stressful moments is one of the most valuable skills you'll ever develop as a nurse.

This chapter will help you understand how to navigate high- pressure situations with clarity, calm, and confidence, even when everything around you feels chaotic.

Stress Is Part of Nursing, But Panic Doesn't Have to Be

Every nurse, no matter how experienced, feels stress. The difference is that experienced nurses have learned how to manage it. They've learned how to pause, breathe, and think clearly, even when the situation is intense.

You will learn this too.

Stress becomes manageable when you:

- Slow down your mind
- Focus on what matters most
- Break tasks into steps

- Lean on your team
- Trust your training

You don't have to eliminate stress; you just have to learn how to move through it.

Pause Before You React

In stressful moments, your instinct may be to rush. But rushing often leads to mistakes. The safest thing you can do is pause, even for a few seconds.

A simple grounding technique is:

- Stop
- Take a breath
- Observe what's happening
- Proceed with intention

This tiny pause helps your brain shift from panic to problem- solving.

Use Your Frameworks When You Feel Overwhelmed

When your mind feels scattered, go back to the basics. Frameworks like ABCs (Airway, Breathing, Circulation) or Maslow's Hierarchy help you quickly identify what needs attention first.

Ask yourself:

- Is the airway open?
- Is the patient breathing normally?
- Is circulation stable?
- Is there immediate danger?

These questions bring clarity when everything feels urgent.

Call for Help Early, Not Late

One of the strongest habits you can build is asking for help as soon as you sense something is wrong. You don't need to wait until you're certain. You don't need to wait until you have all the answers.

If something feels off:

- Call your charge nurse
- Notify the provider
- Ask a coworker to take a look
- Activate rapid response if needed

You are never bothering anyone by advocating for your patient.

Stay Focused on the Patient, Not the Pressure

When a situation becomes stressful, it's easy to get caught up in the noise, the alarms, the voices, and the urgency. But the most important thing is always the patient in front of you.

Ask yourself:

- What does this patient need right now?
- What is the safest next step?
- What can I do in this moment?

Focusing on the patient helps you stay grounded and purposeful.

Use Your Team: You Are Not Alone

Nursing is a team profession. In stressful situations, your team becomes your greatest resource.

You can say:

- "Can you grab vitals while I get the provider on the phone?"
- "Can someone bring the crash cart?"
- "I need another set of eyes on this patient."

Asking for help is not a sign of weakness; it's a sign of safe practice.

Stay Calm on the Outside, Even If You're Shaking on the Inside

Your patients look to you for reassurance. Your calm presence can make a frightening situation feel manageable for them.

You don't need to feel calm to act calm.

You just need to stay steady enough to think clearly.

A calm tone, slow movements, and confident body language help everyone, including you.

Debrief After Stressful Moments

Reflection is essential for growth. After a stressful situation, take a moment to ask yourself:

- What went well?
- What challenged me?
- What did I learn?
- What would I do differently next time?

You can also debrief with your team. These conversations help you process the experience and build confidence for the future.

You Will Get Better at This

Handling stress is not something you master overnight. It's something you grow into, shift by shift, situation by situation.

Over time, you will:

- Recognize early signs of deterioration
- Respond more quickly and calmly
- Communicate more clearly
- Trust your instincts
- Feel more confident in emergencies

You won't always feel comfortable, but you will become capable.

And capability is what truly matters.

You are stronger than you think.

You are learning more than you realize.

And every stressful moment you navigate is shaping you into a more confident, resilient nurse.

Chapter 8 Preventing Burnout Before It Starts

Burnout is one of the most common challenges nurses face, especially new nurses who are still adjusting to the emotional, physical, and mental demands of the profession. You may love your job and still feel exhausted. You may care deeply about your patients and still feel overwhelmed. You may want to grow in your career and still feel drained at the end of the day.

Burnout doesn't happen overnight. It builds slowly, often quietly, through stress, overwork, emotional strain, and the pressure to always be "on." The good news is that burnout can be prevented, and you can build habits now that protect your energy, your passion, and your well- being for years to come.

This chapter will help you understand what burnout looks like, why it happens, and how to protect yourself from it.

Burnout Is Not a Personal Failure

Many nurses feel guilty when they start to feel burned out. They think:

- "Maybe I'm not strong enough."
- "Maybe I'm not cut out for this."
- "Other nurses handle this better than I do."

None of that is true.

Burnout is not a sign of weakness.

Burnout is not a lack of passion.

Burnout is not a reflection of your worth.

Burnout is a natural response to prolonged stress, and it can happen to anyone.

Recognizing it early is a sign of self- awareness, not failure.

Know the Early Signs of Burnout

Burnout rarely starts with dramatic symptoms. It begins with small shifts that are easy to overlook.

Common early signs include:

- Feeling emotionally drained
- Dreading your shifts
- Becoming easily irritated
- Feeling detached from your work
- Trouble sleeping
- Losing interest in things you normally enjoy
- Feeling like you're "running on empty"

If you notice these signs, it's time to pause and take care of yourself.

Set Boundaries and Protect Them

Boundaries are essential in nursing. Without them, you'll give more than you have, and eventually, you'll feel depleted.

Healthy boundaries look like:

- Saying no to extra shifts when you're exhausted
- Leaving work at work

- Not checking your work email or messages on your days off
- Taking your breaks every shift
- Speaking up when your workload is unsafe

You cannot pour from an empty cup. Boundaries help you stay full enough to care for others.

Take Your Breaks; They Are Not Optional

New nurses often skip breaks because they feel guilty or overwhelmed. But breaks are not a luxury; they are a necessity.

Even a 10- minute pause can:

- Lower your stress
- Clear your mind
- Improve your focus
- Prevent mistakes
- Restore your energy

You deserve to eat.

You deserve to hydrate.

You deserve to breathe.

Your patients benefit when you take care of yourself.

Build a Support System

Nursing is too demanding to do alone. You need people who understand the challenges, the emotions, and the realities of the job.

Your support system might include:

- Coworkers you trust
- A mentor or preceptor
- Friends or family
- A therapist or counselor
- Other nurses in online communities

Talking about your experiences helps you process them. You don't have to carry everything by yourself.

Develop Healthy Coping Habits

Coping habits are the tools you use to manage stress. Healthy habits help you recover. Unhealthy habits drain you further.

Healthy coping habits include:

- Exercise or movement
- Journaling
- Prayer or meditation
- Spending time outdoors
- Creative hobbies
- Listening to music
- Resting without guilt

Find what works for you and make it part of your routine.

Give Yourself Permission to Rest

Rest is not laziness. Rest is not weakness. Rest is not unproductive.

Rest is recovery.

Rest is healing.

Rest is necessary.

You cannot be a safe, compassionate nurse if you are constantly running on empty. Rest allows you to show up fully for your patients and for yourself.

Remember Why You Started, But Don't Use It to Pressure Yourself

Your passion for nursing is important, but it should never be used as a reason to push yourself past your limits. You can love your job and still need rest. You can care deeply and still need time away.

Your "why" should inspire you, not exhaust you.

Burnout Prevention Is a Lifelong Practice

Preventing burnout isn't something you do once. It's something you commit to throughout your career. It's a combination of:

- Awareness
- Boundaries
- Self- care
- Support
- Rest
- Reflection

You deserve a long, fulfilling career, not one cut short by exhaustion.

You are allowed to take care of yourself.

You are allowed to rest.

You are allowed to protect your peace.

And doing so will make you a stronger, safer, more compassionate nurse.

Chapter 9 Growing into Your Professional Identity

Becoming a nurse isn't something that happens the day you pass the NCLEX or the day you start your first job. It's a gradual transformation, one that unfolds shift by shift, experience by experience, challenge by challenge. You don't wake up one morning suddenly feeling like a "real nurse." Instead, you grow into your professional identity over time.

This chapter will help you understand what that growth looks like, how to embrace it, and how to continue developing into the nurse you're meant to be.

Your Professional Identity Is Not Defined on Day One

When you're new, it's easy to compare yourself to experienced nurses and feel like you're not measuring up. But the nurse you admire today didn't start out confident, fast, or knowledgeable. They grew into their role, just like you will.

Your professional identity is shaped by:

- Your values
- Your strengths
- Your communication style
- Your approach to patient care
- Your experiences
- Your challenges
- Your growth

You don't need to have everything figured out. You're building your identity one shift at a time.

You Learn Who You Are Through Real Experiences

Nursing school teaches you the foundation. The bedside teaches you who you are as a nurse.

You learn through:

- The first time you advocate for a patient
- The first time you catch a subtle change
- The first time you handle a difficult situation
- The first time you comfort a scared family
- The first time you trust your own judgment

These moments shape you more than any textbook ever could.

Feedback Helps You Grow, Not Shrink

Feedback can feel intimidating, especially when you're new. But feedback is one of the most powerful tools for growth.

Healthy feedback:

- Helps you improve
- Strengthens your skills
- Builds your confidence
- Shows you what you're doing well
- Highlights areas to refine

You are not expected to be perfect. You are expected to learn. And feedback is part of that learning.

Seek Out Mentorship

A mentor doesn't have to be someone formally assigned to you. It can be:

- A nurse you admire
- A coworker who communicates well
- Someone who handles stress gracefully
- A nurse who makes patients feel safe
- Someone who teaches without judgment

Mentors help you:

- Build confidence
- Learn faster
- Avoid common mistakes
- Feel supported
- Grow professionally

You don't have to navigate your first year alone.

Your Strengths Will Become Clearer Over Time

Every nurse has unique strengths. Some are naturally calm. Some are highly organized. Some are great educators. Some are strong advocates. Some are detail- oriented. Some are intuitive.

As you gain experience, you'll start to notice:

- What comes naturally to you
- What energizes you
- What patients appreciate about you
- What coworkers rely on you for

These strengths will shape your identity and guide your career path.

Professional Growth Requires Self- Reflection

Reflection helps you understand your experiences and turn them into growth.

Ask yourself:

- What did I learn today?
- What challenged me?
- What am I proud of?
- What do I want to improve?
- What kind of nurse do I want to become?

Reflection turns experience into wisdom.

You Don't Have to Rush Your Growth

There is no timeline for becoming a confident nurse. Some nurses feel comfortable after six months. Others take a year or more. Both are normal.

Growth is not a race.

Growth is not linear.

Growth is not something you can force.

You grow by showing up, learning, asking questions, and caring deeply.

You Are Becoming the Nurse You Once Hoped You'd Be

You may not see it yet, but you are changing. You are learning. You are becoming stronger, more capable, and more confident. You are building a professional identity rooted in compassion, safety, and integrity.

One day, you'll look back and realize:

- You trust your judgment
- You communicate clearly
- You advocate confidently
- You handle challenges with grace

- You are someone others look up to

You are becoming that nurse, slowly, steadily, beautifully.

Your professional identity is not something you find.

It's something you grow into.

And you're already on your way.

Chapter 10 Becoming the Nurse You're Meant to Be

There will come a moment, maybe months from now, maybe a year, when you'll pause in the middle of a shift and realize something has changed. You'll notice that your hands move with more confidence. Your voice sounds steadier. Your decisions feel clearer. You'll catch yourself comforting a patient with ease, advocating without hesitation, or handling a situation that once would have overwhelmed you.

And in that moment, you'll understand something important:

You've grown.

Not all at once. Not overnight. But steadily, quietly, beautifully; shift by shift, patient by patient, challenge by challenge.

This final chapter is a reminder of who you are becoming and why your journey matters.

You Are Stronger Than You Realize

Nursing will test you. It will stretch you. It will push you into moments you never imagined you could handle. But every time you rise to the challenge, even when you feel scared, unsure, or exhausted, you prove something to yourself.

You are stronger than you think.

You are more capable than you believe.

You are growing in ways you can't always see.

Strength isn't loud. Strength isn't perfect. Strength is showing up, caring deeply, and doing your best even on hard days.

You Are Making a Difference

You may not always see the impact you have, but it's there.

It's in the patient who feels safe because you took the time to explain their medication.

It's in the family member who feels comforted because you listened without rushing.

It's in the subtle change you caught that prevented a complication.

It's in the coworker who feels supported because you stepped in to help.

Nursing is full of quiet victories, the kind that don't get announced but matter deeply.

You are part of those victories.

You are part of someone's healing.

You are part of someone's hope.

You Are Allowed to Grow at Your Own Pace

There is no single timeline for becoming a confident nurse. Some nurses find their rhythm quickly. Others take longer. Both paths are valid.

Growth is not a race.

Growth is not linear.

Growth is not something you can rush.

You are allowed to learn slowly.

You are allowed to ask questions.

You are allowed to make mistakes and grow from them.

Your journey is your own, and it's unfolding exactly as it should.

You Are Building a Career with Purpose

Nursing is more than a job. It's a calling, a responsibility, and a privilege. You are entering a profession built on compassion, integrity, and service. A profession that asks a lot from you but also gives you moments of meaning that stay with you forever.

As you grow, you'll discover:

- What kind of nurse do you want to be
- What areas of practice inspire you
- What strengths define you
- What values guide your care

Your career will evolve, and so will you. And that evolution is something to embrace, not fear.

You Are Becoming the Nurse You Once Needed

Think back to the version of yourself who walked into the hospital on your first day: nervous, unsure, overwhelmed, but hopeful. That version of you needed guidance, reassurance, and support.

And now, slowly but surely, you are becoming that person for someone else.

One day, a new nurse will look at you the way you once looked at others, with admiration, with trust, with the belief that you know what you're doing. And you will. Because you've earned it.

Your Journey Doesn't End Here; It Begins Here

This book is not the end of your growth. It's the beginning of a long, meaningful, fulfilling career. You will continue to learn, adapt, and evolve. You will face challenges, but you will also experience moments of joy, pride, and purpose that remind you why you chose this path.

You are not expected to be perfect.

You are expected to care.

You are expected to grow.

You are expected to keep showing up.

And you will.

Because you are becoming the nurse you're meant to be—one shift at a time, one patient at a time, one moment at a time.

Closing Thoughts

You're Growing More Than You Realize

As you reach the end of this book, I want you to pause for a moment and recognize something important: the very fact that you're here—reading, learning, reflecting, seeking guidance—is proof of your dedication and your heart. It shows that you care deeply about becoming the best nurse you can be. And that alone sets you apart.

Your first year will not always be easy. There will be days that test you, moments that overwhelm you, and shifts that leave you questioning everything. But there will also be moments of connection, gratitude, growth, and quiet triumph. Moments when you realize you made a difference. Moments when you feel yourself becoming stronger, steadier, and more confident.

You won't always see your growth as it's happening. But it's there in the way you speak up, the way you advocate, the way you think through problems, the way you show compassion even when you're tired. Growth is not loud. It's not dramatic. It's steady, patient, and persistent.

And you are growing.

My hope is that this book becomes a companion you return to on the hard days, on the uncertain days, and even on the good days when you simply want to remember how far you've come. You are not alone in this journey. You never were.

You are becoming the nurse you're meant to be.

And I'm cheering for you every step of the way.

About the Author

Alice Ashu, BSN, RN, is a dedicated registered nurse whose journey as a nurse began far from where she stands today. Born and raised in a small community, she immigrated to the United States with big dreams and an even bigger heart. Nursing became the place where her compassion, resilience, and quiet strength found their purpose.

Her early years in nursing were shaped by mentors who believed in her before she believed in herself, patients who taught her the true meaning of care, and experiences that revealed the power of calmness, softness, and empathy in a fast- paced medical world. She learned that confidence isn't something you start with; it's something you grow into.

Today, she uses her voice to uplift and guide new nurses who feel the same uncertainty she once felt. Through her writing, she offers the support, reassurance, and practical wisdom she wished she had during her first year.

Her mission is simple:

To remind every new nurse that they are capable, they are growing, and that they belong.

When she's not caring for patients or writing, she enjoys quiet moments, meaningful conversations, and the joy of watching others discover their own strength.